HOW TO APPLY GUA SHA FOR BEGINNERS

Ultimate beginners guide on how to apply gua sha, uses, benefits, symptoms and how to utilize it

Table of Contents

CHAPTER ONE 3

    INTRODUCTION 3

    MEANING OF GUA SHA 4

CHAPTER TWO 11

    USES OF GUA SHA 11

    BENEFITS OF USING GUA SHA 12

    SYMPTOMS AND DANGERS..............................14

    GUA SHA EQUIPMENT AND METHOD............17

CHAPTER THREE 19

    GUA SHA VARIATIONS.....................................19

    HOW TO USE GUA SHA 22

    UTILIZING GUA SHA...26

    USING GUA SHA ON YOUR FACE 26

CHAPTER FOUR 30

    STEPS ON HOW TO USE GUA SHA STONES 30

    SYMPTOMS OF PERIMENOPAUSE 35

    AID IN REDUCING DIABETIC NEUROPATHY 37

    ATHLETIC PERFORMANCE AND RECOVERY 39

    TREAT AUTOIMMUNE DISORDERS.............40

THE END 42

CHAPTER ONE

INTRODUCTION

A method called gua sha is employed in conventional East Asian medicine. Although there has not been much research on how well it works, it is frequently used to treat muscle pain and tension. Gua sha attempts to circulate the body's qi or chi energy. The procedure involves rubbing the skin with a tool in long strokes while exerting just enough pressure to cause light bruises. Gua sha may facilitate the breakdown of connective tissue and scar tissue, enhancing joint mobility. Although there are no severe side effects from the treatment, some medical conditions prevent some people from receiving it.

MEANING OF GUA SHA

Gua sha can dissolve scar tissue and be used to treat muscle pain. Gua sha is the practice of applying pressure to the skin and scraping it to release tension and pain. This action results in minor bruising, which frequently takes the form of petechiae or sha, which are red or purple spots the Chinese word for scraping is where the name gua sha, pronounced gwahshah, originates. Other names for it include coining, spooning, and skin scraping. Qi or chi is energy, according to traditional Chinese medicine, that moves throughout the body. Many people think that for someone to be healthy and happy, their qi needs to be balanced and flowing freely. People also think that when qi is blocked, it can lead to muscle and joint pain or tension. Gua sha seeks to release this stagnated energy to ease pain or stiffness. Blood stasis or stagnation is another factor that traditional East Asian medicine believes contributes to pain and illness. Gua sha's ability to move blood that has accumulated or stagnated is another goal. Instrument assisted soft tissue mobilization is a variation of the technique that some physiotherapists employ (IASTM). A physiotherapist can exert more pressure during a massage by using a tool rather than their hands.

One of the fastest and most efficient ways to lift, sculpt, and contour your face is with facial gua sha. The exercise promotes stronger facial muscles, improved skin texture and elasticity, reduced puffiness, healthier skin tissue, and improved circulation when it is performed correctly and on a regular basis. You will have a more youthful, toned complexion with a natural glow if your skin changes in this way. Gua sha will improve your skin's overall functionality and slow down the aging process by boosting circulation and encouraging healthy lymphatic flow. I advise practicing gua sha in the direction of lymph flow, beginning on your neck and briskly working your way up, just like facial massage. This can eventually improve other underlying conditions like acne, pigmentation, and rosacea by clearing out stagnant energy and toxin buildup. Before focusing on the area around your face, I think it's crucial to fully open up the neck with your tool. The neck is in charge of how your face is moving. Because there are numerous lymph nodes in the neck region, take your time and be gentle. You can skip your face and focus solely on your neck if you have a breakout or any other skin issues on your face. If the condition doesn't change or clear up, you can continue your routine by concentrating on the neck and returning to the face later. You want facial gua sha to be a soothing procedure. Move slowly, take deep breaths, and most importantly, drink plenty of water. This ritual can be performed daily or two to three times per week in the morning or evening. Use each movement 5–10 times per area for the best results. I advise doing it earlier in the day so you can concentrate on staying hydrated and continuing to drink lots of water after. Because it makes me feel and look more awake, I prefer the mornings. Your appearance and mood change as you incorporate this more into your daily skincare regimen. It's crucial to get your skin ready for gua sha. Make sure your skin is entirely clean. To make your tool glide more easily, apply an oil, balm, or lotion. Although I prefer oil, you should use whatever is best for your skin and won't irritate or cause a breakout. Make sure your product is nutrient-rich and non-toxic to aid in promoting lymphatic flow. A hydration mist is an additional option. There's no doubt that you've heard of gua sha, the tiny flat pebble renowned for its ability to chisel out cheekbones you didn't know you had if you're a fan of skincare rollers and tools. It's a traditional Chinese technique that is pronounced "gwah-sha" and is intended to increase blood flow, reduce stress, and improve circulation. This can be compared to a trifecta of self-care, massage, and skincare. The sandy dark spots that appear on the skin after a gua sha body treatment are referred to by the literal translation of the words "gua" and "sha," which is "sand," Although gua sha can be applied to any part of the body, facial gua sha is currently very popular. Even though the movements are very light and there isn't any actual scraping or pressure used, the technique results in skin that is more sculpted and toned and has a glowing complexion.

CHAPTER TWO

USES OF GUA SHA

The most frequent uses of gua sha are to treat joint and muscle pain. Musculoskeletal disorders are conditions affecting the muscles and bones. Back pain, tendonitis, and carpal tunnel syndrome are a few examples. Gua sha practitioners assert that it can strengthen the immune system and lessen inflammation. Gua sha can occasionally be used to treat respiratory issues, fevers, and colds. Micro trauma is the term for minor bodily wounds, such as the bruises brought on by gua sha. These trigger a reaction in the body that could aid in reducing scar tissue. Fibrosis, which results from an excess buildup of connective tissue during the healing process, may also be helped by micro trauma. IASTM can be applied by physiotherapists to connective tissue that isn't moving joints properly. A repetitive strain injury or another condition could be to blame for this issue. Along with other therapies like stretching and strengthening exercises, gua sha is used.

BENEFITS OF USING GUA SHA

According to studies, gua sha may be beneficial for those who use computers and experience neck and shoulder pain. To determine whether gua sha is effective, researchers have conducted small studies on the following populations:

1. Older people with back pain

2. Women who are approaching menopause

3. Computer users' neck and shoulders

4. Male weightlifters to aid in recovery after training

Women discovered that after gua sha, per menopause symptoms like sweating, insomnia, and headaches were lessened. In comparison to a control group that received no treatment, gua sha improved range of motion and decreased pain in people who frequently use computers.

In a 2017 study, weightlifters who received gua sha reported that it was easier to lift weights after the procedure. This may indicate that the medication hastens muscle recovery. Both gua sha and a hot pack were used to treat older adults who had back pain. Both treatments effectively reduced symptoms, In comparison to the control group, those who had received gua sha treatment reported more flexibility and less back pain after a week.

SYMPTOMS AND DANGERS

Capillaries, which are tiny blood vessels close to the skin's surface, rupture as a result of gua sha. Sha, or distinctive red or purple bruises, are the result of this.

The bruises can be tender while healing and typically take a few days or a week to disappear. To ease pain and reduce swelling, people can take an over-the-counter painkiller like ibuprofen. A person should be careful not to bump the bruised area and protect it. An ice pack can be used to reduce swelling and ease any pain. Although gua sha practitioners are advised not to break the skin during the procedure, it is possible. A gua sha reduces the risk of infection by healing broken skin. Between procedures, the practitioner should always sterilize their equipment. Not everyone is a good candidate for gua sha. A person should not receive gua sha if they are:

1. Who suffer from illnesses that affect their veins or skin.

2. Those that are prone to bleeding easily take blood-thinning medication have deep vein thrombosis, an infection, a tumor, or an open wound that hasn't fully recovered, as well as those who have implants like a pacemaker or internal defibrillator.

Gua sha is it painful?

Treatments are not supposed to hurt, but gua sha purposefully bruises, which some people may find uncomfortable. Within a few days, these bruises should disappear.

GUA SHA EQUIPMENT AND METHOD

Gua sha is performed with a hand-held tool that has rounded edges. Modern therapists scrape the skin with a small, hand-held tool with rounded edges rather than the conventional spoon or coin. Tools used in gua sha are frequently weighted to make it easier for the practitioner performing the procedure to apply pressure. Traditional East Asian medicine practitioners believe that certain objects, such as rose quartz, jade, and bian stone, have an energy that promotes healing. For IASTM or when gua sha is performed in a clinic, medical grade stainless steel is frequently utilized.

To help the therapist move the tool across the skin more smoothly, practitioners will apply oil to the area of the body that is being treated. The gua sha practitioner will apply firm, fluid strokes in one direction to the body. A person may need to lie face down on a massage table if gua sha is being performed on the back or backs of the legs.

CHAPTER THREE

GUA SHA VARIATIONS

Gua sha tools are available in a wide range of sizes and shapes to fit various body and facial regions. "Heart shapes, moon shapes, and various iterations of rectangular shapes are gua sha tools. For various parts of the face, some have concaves, pointed edges, curly curved edges, and comb edges. There are also gua shas designed for specific, specialized purposes, such as the knobbed-appearing "mushroom" gua shas for the eye region and the longer, stick-like acupressure gua shas. All tools have gently rounded edges that won't irritate skin. You'll notice that gua sha tools come in a variety of shapes and materials, including rose quartz, turquoise, jade, obsidian, glass, and even wood. The concept is that every stone has a particular healing function. Each material can benefit our body with different energetic and therapeutic properties, so when you choose a gua sha tool for yourself, choose one according to your needs. Benefits of Gua Sha Advocates of gua sha concur that the practice has both physical and mental advantages. Gua sha brightens your complexion, contours and sculpts, and softens wrinkles and fine lines." Some claim that it can also ease sinus pressure, headaches, and TMJ pain. Gua sha tools can be helpful in reducing inflammation and puffiness by compression facial massage."

"Additionally, it can aid in the microcirculation of lymphatic drainage in the facial cosmetic subunits. As interstitial fluid can collect in these areas overnight when laying flat, this is particularly true for the under eye area in the morning to reduce puffiness. There are mental advantages as well "Any form of self-care, in my opinion, can serve as a ritual for you. Gua sha feels grounding to my spirit and promotes inner self-care for me. When I incorporate the ritual into my skincare routine, I feel balanced because I am breathing through the techniques and clearing my mind.

HOW TO USE GUA SHA

Are you prepared to master the use of your gua sha tool? It's a fairly easy process that anyone can complete.

Tone and Cleanse

Gua sha should only be applied to clean skin. Apply toner if using it after cleansing. Additionally, make sure the tool is clean as well as your hands. You only need a drop of cleanser and some water.

Apply facial oil

Apply plenty of face oil to your chest, neck, and face. However, if you prefer a cream or water-based lotion, that is acceptable as well. Oil will make the tool glide more easily. Just be aware that you might need to apply more times as the process progresses. Practice Gua Sha At this point, you can start your actual practice of gua sha. Pull or scrape the tool across your skin very gently while holding it at a 30 to 45 degree angle. Every movement should generally be upward and follow lymphatic flow. Before tackling the next area of your skin, repeat each motion three to five times. The following movements should be incorporated into your gua sha facial routine, according to Campbell-Semien:

1. **Chin and jaw line:** To shape the jaw, move your tool from the chin's center out toward the earlobe.

2. **Forehead:** Glide your tool outward starting in the middle of your forehead, and then divide it into three sections. Scrape once, then descend a little and scrape once more.

3. **Cheek:** Beginning at the nose, move outwards toward your ears while sweeping upward along the cheeks and cheekbones. Move down a little, scrape once more, then move to the center of the chin and scrape once more.

4. **under eye:** Work from the inner corner of the eye to the temple.

5. **Brows:** From the inside out, gently glide upward along the brow bone.

6. Lips: For a plumping effect, glide over your lips five times back and forth.

7. **Neck:** Divide your neck into four sections, and then scrape each one starting at the bottom.

Eliminate Extras and Finish the Regimen

If you choose, you can use your hands to massage the remaining product into your skin or a damp cloth to remove any remaining oil or cream. After that, finish your usual skincare routine. practicing gua sha three to four times a week for between three and five minutes each time, for best results.

UTILIZING GUA SHA

Gua sha is performed by simply gliding one of the tools' smooth edges across the skin twice while applying light pressure. Before using the tool, you could treat the area with a cream or serum to make it glide more easily. However, "People with sensitive skin may want to avoid gua sha because excessive pressure can cause skin irritation. Although there aren't many side effects, applying too much pressure can make it uncomfortable and cause bruising or soreness.

USING GUA SHA ON YOUR FACE

it is best to use gua sha on your face in the morning when you are at your puffiest.

1.   **Neck:** Sweep the wide side of the tool upward to your jaw line while starting from your right collarbone. you should hold a gua sha tool at a very slight angle, nearly parallel to your skin. They actually cut into the meridians like a knife would through bread. In Chinese medicine, you try to move in conjunction with the meridians to encourage them to open.

2.   Applying "light and gentle" pressure. The face has a very intelligent system, so when you hit it too hard, the meridians will actually close to protect themselves, according to the expert.

3.   Move to your face after starting with your neck.

4.   You should begin a session at your neck and work your way up. The neck and chest need to be released first and foremost, "I think a lot of people want to go straight to the face because they think that's where they're trying to get the results," she says. "Since the neck serves as a connection between the face and the body, it will aid in circulation. You won't get a good result on your face if you skip over your neck because it is so tight. Strong neck muscles may pull the face downward, resulting in a droopy appearance or a dejected expression. "

5.   Depending on how you feel, you can use a gua sha tool as frequently or infrequently as you like, choosing short or

lengthy sessions. This practice has beauty. It accepts you exactly as you are.

CHAPTER FOUR

STEPS ON HOW TO USE GUA SHA STONES

1. From your collarbone to your earlobe, sweep the gua sha tool up your neck.

2. Repeat up to your chin, closer to the middle of your neck.

3. Jaw line

4. Along your jaw line, move the gua sha tool under your chin and toward your earlobe.

5. To loosen up the jaw, gently wiggle the tool's end.

6. Cheek 1. Sweep the tool underneath your cheekbone, toward your hairline to

collect stagnant fluid and energy. Sweep it along your jaw line from the corner of your mouth up to your earlobe.

7.   under Eye 1. Quickly flick the gua sha stone from under your eye to your temple.

8. Sweep the tool up from the brow bone and over your eyebrow, out toward your hairline sweeping it up your forehead.

9. Move the tool from the space between your brows up to the hairline, passing over the third eye, which is situated in the center of your forehead.

10.   Sweep the gua sha tool horizontally across your forehead, starting in the center and ending at your hairline.

11. Move the gua sha tool along your jawline, under your chin, and toward your earlobe.

12. To loosen up the jaw, gently wiggle the tool's end.

13. Sweep it up to your earlobe from the bottom of your chin, beginning at the corner of your mouth.

14. Cheek 1. To remove stagnant fluid and energy, sweep the tool beneath your cheekbone in the direction of your hairline.

15. under Eye 1. Quickly flick the gua sha stone from under your eye to your temple.

16. Sweep the tool up from the brow bone and over your eyebrow, out toward your hairline sweeping it up your forehead.

17. Move the tool from the space between your brows up to the hairline, passing over the third eye, which is situated in the center of your forehead.

18. Sweep the gua sha tool horizontally across your forehead, starting in the center and ending at your hairline.

19. Gua Sha's Potential Health Benefits May Help with Chronic Pain

20. Gua sha encourages blood flow to the area being scraped, which can help lessen pain and stiffness. It's frequently used to treat swelling, neck and back pain, and tension headaches.

21. In fact, the Graston Technique, which is a technique similar to gua sha, is

frequently used by physical therapists to lessen pain and increase mobility in patients with musculoskeletal conditions.

22. Gua sha on the shoulder can break down microscopic scar tissue or adhesions if someone has adhesive capsulitis, also known as frozen shoulder. Scraping increases range of motion and reduces pain by mobilizing the tissue, enhancing circulation, and thinning out muscle knots.

23. In a previous study, for instance, adults with chronic neck pain who underwent a single gua sha treatment experienced significantly less pain after a week as compared to those who used a heating pad. However, more research is required to determine whether gua sha is

effective in the long-term management of neck pain.

24. Comparatively to the control group, patients with chronic lower back pain reported lower pain intensity and better overall health after two gua sha treatments.

SYMPTOMS OF PERIMENOPAUSE

perimenopause is the period between menopause and the end of a woman's reproductive years. Many women who experience it have hot flashes, sleep issues, and mood swings as physical symptoms. Menopausal symptoms can be treated in a variety of ways, but some women choose complementary therapies like gua sha, under the supervision of a healthcare professional, to develop an integrative strategy for managing the perimenopause transition. Women with perimenopause symptoms who additionally received weekly 15-minute gua sha treatments saw more pronounced improvements in their symptoms and quality of life than those who did not. After eight weeks, the women in the gua sha group specifically reported greater decreases in hot flashes, insomnia, fatigue, nervousness, and headache. Gua sha may be a promising, efficient, non-drug treatment for perimenopausal syndrome in some women, though more research is required.

AID IN REDUCING DIABETIC NEUROPATHY

Diabetic neuropathy is a serious diabetes complication that can affect up to 50% of diabetics. It is a form of nerve damage that happens when high blood sugar glucose levels harm nerves all over the body. Diabetic neuropathy can cause issues with the heart, digestive system, urinary tract, blood vessels, and feet in addition to the usual numbness and pain in the legs and feet. Gua sha may be beneficial by increasing circulation and improving nerve conduction. Patients with diabetic neuropathy experienced significant symptom improvements after 12 weekly gua sha sessions in a randomized controlled trial conducted in China and published in Complementary Therapies in Clinical Practice in 2019 as opposed to those who did not receive gua sha. The patients stated that their sensory function, balance, nighttime burning in their legs and feet, and plasma glucose levels had all improved a common method of diagnosing and monitoring diabetes. Given the paucity of research, it's probably best that you continue receiving standard diabetes and neurology care for the time being. Before attempting gua sha as a complementary therapy, speak with your doctor.

ATHLETIC PERFORMANCE AND RECOVERY

Gua sha may enhance exercise performance and hasten recovery afterward. Men were given gua sha, sham gua sha (no petechiae), or no gua sha in a study that was published in the Journal of Traditional Chinese Medicine in 2019 along with their regular twice-weekly weightlifting workouts. Even though everyone used only 85% of their one-rep max the most weight they can lift in one repetition, the men who received gua sha after eight weeks of therapy reported less perceived effort in completing the snatch and clean and jerk exercise than the other men. The fact that the men weren't constrained by fatigue from prior training sessions led researchers to hypothesize that gua sha may have promoted faster muscle recovery. These outcomes confirm those of a study that was reported in the Journal of Traditional Chinese Medicine in 2017. Larger studies, though, are required to validate these findings.

TREAT AUTOIMMUNE DISORDERS

Gua sha may help those with autoimmune diseases, despite the paucity of research in this area. You can use gua sha to reduce systemic inflammation, so I use it a lot on patients with autoimmune diseases, like lupus." Continually doing it could help reduce inflammation and ease symptoms, Scraping the tissues helps the body's blood and nutrients circulate more effectively, which can reduce inflammation. Stimulating petechiae may also activate the anti-inflammatory immune proteins known as cytokines. Always check with your primary healthcare provider before attempting any new complementary therapies, and remember that gua sha is not a cure for autoimmune diseases. To fully comprehend how gua sha might benefit those with autoimmune diseases, more study is still required.

THE END